Longevity Training-Book1-Long Lived Persons

Copyright Page

The book is copyrighted for 2018

Longevity Training-Book 1-Long Lived People

By Martin K. Ettington

All Rights Reserved USA 2018

ISBN: 9781729073506

Printed in the United States of America

Longevity Training-Book1-Long Lived Persons

Longevity Training-Book1-Long Lived Persons

This book is a transcription and reproduction of the training course materials from Course #1 Long Lived Persons from the Longevity Coaching Training Server.

Except for being printed instead of Audio/Visual, it is the same content presented in that course.

The first course and this book is designed to give you a full introduction into the in depth exploration of Long Lived People and Myths about even longer lived people.

My objective is that after you have read this material you will truly understand the reality of long lived people really existing in this world.

If you are going to learn how to live decades longer than the normal life expectancy, then knowing it is really possible and has been done before is the first great step.

Longevity Training-Book1-Long Lived Persons

Longevity Training-Book1-Long Lived Persons

Other books by Martin K. Ettington

<u>Spiritual and Metaphysics Books:</u>
Prophecy: A History and How to Guide
God Like Powers and Abilities
Enlightenment for Newbies
Removing Illusions to Find True
    Happiness
Using the Scientific Method to Study
    the Paranormal
A Compendium of Metaphysics and
    How to Guides (Six books
    together in one volume)
Love from the Heart
The Enlightenment Experience
Learn Your Soul's Purpose
Pursuing Enlightenment
A Modern Man's Search for Truth
Use Intuition and Prophecy to Improve
    Your Life
The Handbook of Spiritual and Energy
    Healing

<u>Longevity & Immortality:</u>
Physical Immortality: A History and
    How to Guide
The Commentaries of Living Immortals
Records of Extremely Long Lived
    Persons
Enlightenment and Immortality
Longevity Improvements from Science
The 10 Principles of Personal
    Longevity
Telomeres & Longevity
The Diets and Lifestyles of the Worlds
    Oldest Peoples
The Longevity Six Books Bundle

<u>Science Fiction:</u>
Out of This Universe
Personal Freedom-Parts 1 & 2
The Psychic Soldier Series:
    Book 1-Himalayan Journey
    Book 2-A Soldier is Born
    Book 3-Fighting For Right
    Book 4-Earth Protector
The Immortality Sci Fi Bundle

<u>The God Like Powers Series:</u>
Human Invisibility
Invulnerability and Shielding
Teleportation
Psychokinesis
Our Energy Body, Auras, and
Thoughtforms

The God Like Powers Series—
    Volume 1 Compilation
<u>The Yoga Discovery Series:</u>
Yoga-An Ancient Art Form
Hatha Yoga-Helping you Live Better
Raja Yoga-Through the Ages
The Yoga Discovery Package

<u>Business & Coaching Books:</u>
Creating, Paublishing, & Marketing
    Practitioner Ebooks
Building a Successful Longevity
    Coaching Business
Why Become a Coach?
The Professional Coaching Success
Trilogy
2020-Make Money Writing and Selling
    Books
The 2020 Handbook of High Paying
    Work Without a College Degree

<u>Science, Technology, and Misc.</u>
Future Predictions By and Engineer &
    Seer
The Unusual Science & Technology
    Bundle
The Real Atlantis-In the Eye of the
    Sahara
Are Cryptozoological Animals Real or
    Imaginary?
Real Time Travel Stories From a
    Psychic Engineer
Removing Limits On Our
    Consciousness-And
    Thinking Outside the Box
33 Incredible True Survival Stories
How to Survive Anything: From the
    Wilderness to Man Made
    Disasters
All About Mars Journeys and
    Settlement
Mining the Asteroid Belt

<u>Ancient History</u>
The Real Atlantis-In the Eye of the
Sahara
Ancient & Prehistoric Civilizations
Ancient & Prehistoric Civilizations-Book
    Two
The History of Antediluvian Giants
The Antediluvian History of Earth
Ancient Underground Cities and
    Tunnels
Strange Objects Which Should Not Exist

Longevity Training-Book1-Long Lived Persons

Strange and Ancient Places in the USA
A Theory of Ancient Prehistory And
      Giant Aliens
<u>Aliens and Space</u>
Aliens and Secret Technology
Aliens Are Already Among Us
Designing and Building Space Colonies
Humanity and the Universe

All About Moon Bases
All About Mars Journeys and Settlement
The Space and Aliens Six Books Bundle
A Theory of Ancient Prehistory and
      Giant Aliens
The Space Colonies and Space
      Structures Coloring Book
All About Asteroids

<u>The Longevity Training Series</u>

(A transcription of the online Multimedia Longevity Coaching Training Program)

The Personal Longevity Training Series-Book1-Long Lived Persons
The Personal Longevity Training Series-Book2-Your Soul's Purpose
The Personal Longevity Training Series-Book3-Enable Your Life Urge
The Personal Longevity Training Series-Book4-Your Spiritual Connection
The Personal Longevity Training Series-Book5-Having Love in Your Heart
The Personal Longevity Training Series-Book6-Energy Body Health
The Personal Longevity Training Series-Book7-The Science of Longevity
The Personal Longevity Training Series-Book8-Physical Body Health
The Personal Longevity Training Series-Book9-Avoiding Accidents
The Personal Longevity Training Series-Book10-Implementing These Principles

The Personal Longevity Training Series-Books One Thru Ten

These books are all available in digital and printed formats from my
website and on Amazon, Barnes & Noble, Apple ITunes, and many other sites

My Books Website is: http://mkettingtonbooks.com

Longevity Training-Book1-Long Lived Persons

<u>Signup for our Mailing List to get the following:</u>

1) A discount coupon for 25% discount on all books on our site

2) Occasional Notices of new books available

3) Occasional Email on other offerings of ours (Monthly)

Go to this link to sign-up:

http://personal-longevity.com/mkebooks/emailsignup/

And click this link to get the FREE 102 page Ebook titled "Secrets of Many Things"

If you have any questions about this book or other subjects please contact the Author at:

mke@mkettingtonbooks.com

Longevity Training-Book1-Long Lived Persons

Longevity Training-Book1-Long Lived Persons

Longevity Training-Book1-Long Lived Persons

Table of Contents

Longevity Training-Book1-Long Lived Persons

Longevity Training-Book1-Long Lived Persons

Introduction

Back in 2008 I became very interested in the field of Longevity and Physical Immortality. After a lot of research this led me to my first book on the subject "Physical Immortality: A History and How to Guide". This book was pretty popular and I wanted to continue learning about Longevity and what things we could do about it in our lives.

The subject continued to fascinate me to the point that I developed a Longevity Coaching program over a couple of years starting in 2011. This online training program was multimedia—consisting of videos, my writings on longevity to read, online exercises, and tests for each of ten courses. It also included a lot of additional resources for each course including extra courses on how to become a successful Longevity Coach. A student who completed the training and tests successfully would become certified as a "Longevity Coach" and authorized to teach this material to others.

I developed a set of ten principles on longevity which are as follows:

The 10 Principles of Personal Longevity are:

- The Reality of Long Lived People
- Defining Your Purpose in Life
- Enabling the Life Urge
- Your Spiritual Health
- Having Love in Your Heart
- Energy Body Health
- The Science of Longevity
- Physical Body Health
- Using your Intuition for Safety
- Implementation of these principles

What are the 10 Principles all about?

The Reality of Long Lived People

The first principle is where I provide lots of evidence of people who have lived well over the age of 120 years old to 150-180-200, and even a 256 year old man from China:

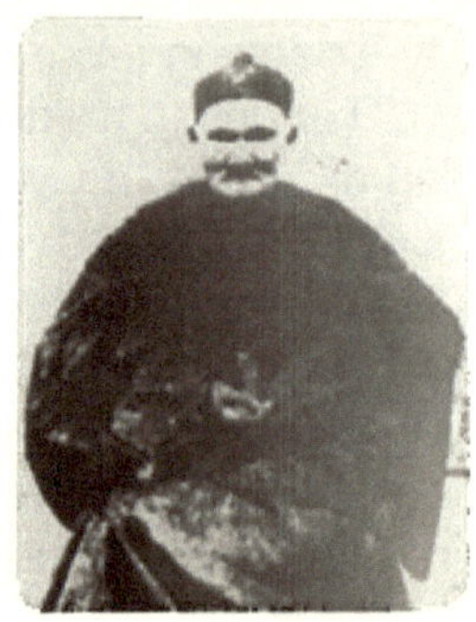

LI CHING-YUN: The Longest Lived person of record-256 Years (Source-The New York Times-May 6, 1933)

The Second Principle of Life Purpose

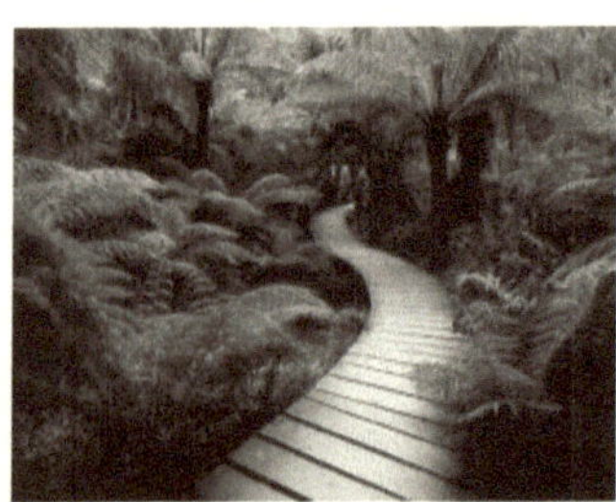

One of the things that occurred to me when I was putting the 10 principles together was that if one doesn't have a reason to live, or purpose in life--then what is the point?

This meant I had to add a very important step of how you can develop your own life purpose, or bring it up to date with your phase in life. Without reviewing your purpose-- then none of the rest of the principles matter.

Enabling the Life Urge

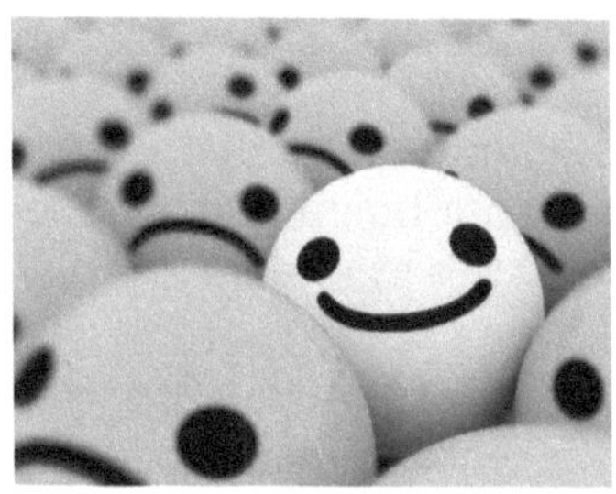

Have you ever realized how we are all programmed to expect to live through certain stages in life and then die? It's so common in our society that we don't think it odd that we expect to die at a certain age?

Have you ever heard radio ads saying "You are getting up in your sixties and seventies" so it's time to come out to our cemetery and buy a plot"

How ridiculous is this? And do you see how much our subconscious has been programmed towards death?

This principle is all about reprogramming ourselves to have a more positive outlook on life and its possibilities.

Having a Spiritual Connection in Your Life

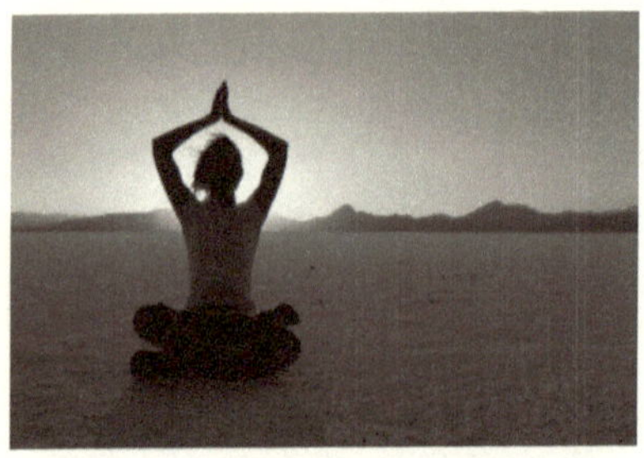

Most of us innately understand that we have a spiritual core in the center of our being. It is this spiritual core that we need to connect with to enable our physical health too.

It doesn't matter what religion you are. Regular meditation, deep prayer, or just walking in the woods helps you make and keep that connection in your life.

Having Love in Your Heart

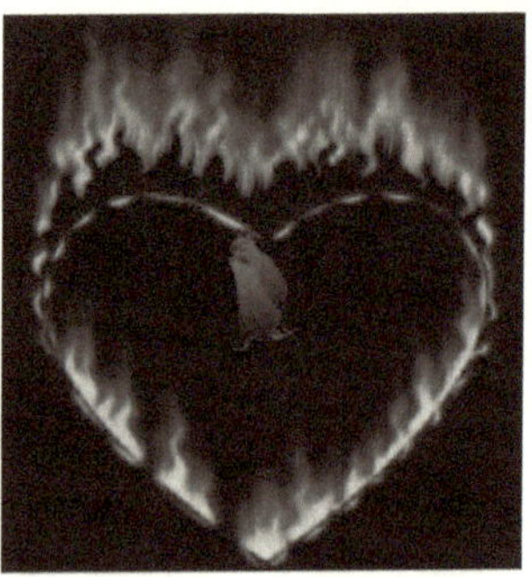

One of the most important things I learned in the last five years was that Unconditional Love is a real and physical thing. It is a powerful energy force in life and not just a philosophical belief system.

I considered it so important that I added it as a separate principle of longevity.

True Unconditional Love is healing, embodies happiness, and is a powerful part of our vital forces.

Energy Body Health

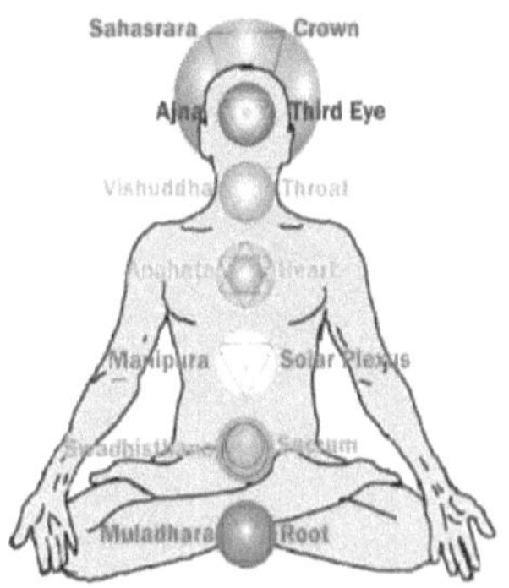

We all have an energy body which is part of our vital forces. The Indians talk about the "Chakras" and the Chinese talk about "Energy Meridians" in Acupuncture.

We should all learn different practices to keep our vital forces flowing for maximum health and vitality.

The Science of Longevity

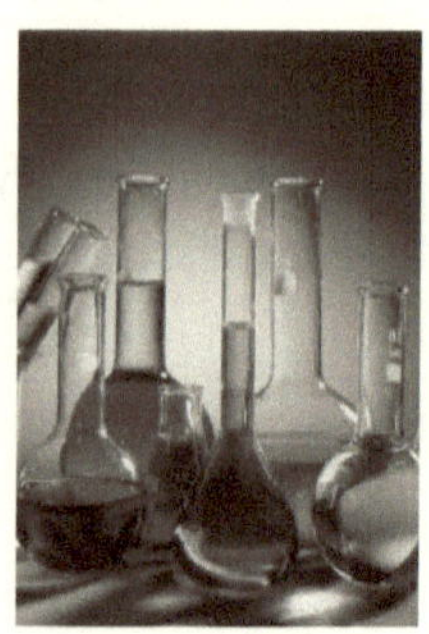

Science and Medicine are making new discoveries all the time that we can take advantage of to extend our lives. Why not take advantage of these discoveries which provide new therapies and supplements to increase our longevity.

There is also a lot we can learn from plants and animals. We all share the same genetic basis.

Some of these plants and animals live thousands of years and some cells are immortal.

What can we learn from them to apply to our lives?

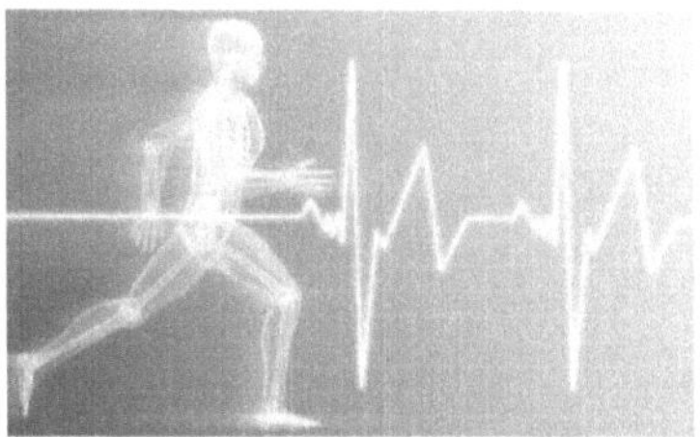

There are many types of supplements used for anti-aging for thousands of years. What can we learn about them that we can apply to our lives?

What other considerations about our physical health does nontraditional or alternative medicine offer?

Using Your Intuition for Safety

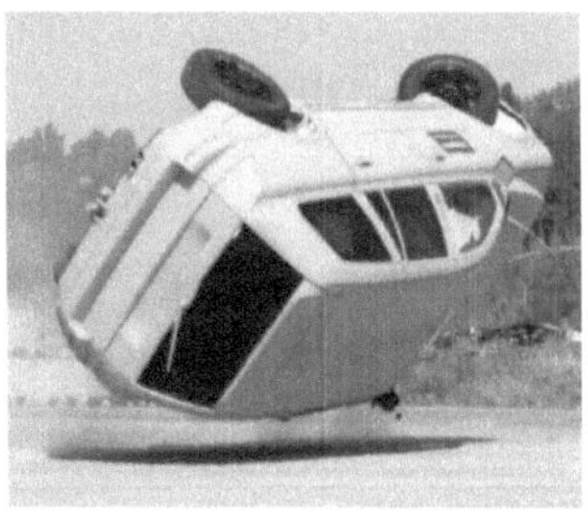

Once you have established your own long term health then what is the greatest danger you face?

ACCIDENTS

We can learn to use our intuition to make us safer as well as see potential future events which may be good too.

Why not open up to the possibilities of how our spirit has this natural ability in all of us?

Implementing These Principles in Your Life

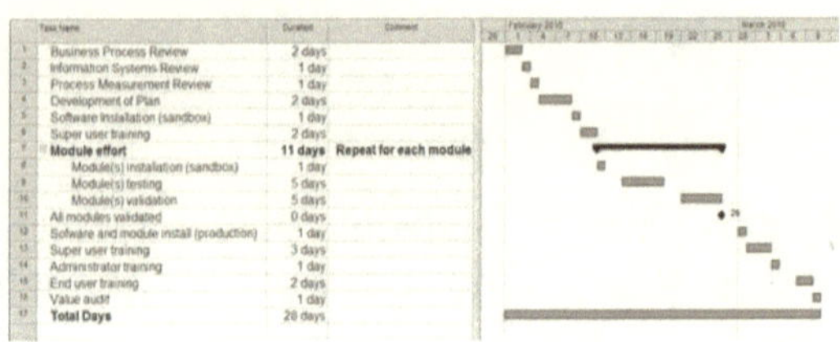

It's nice to read about all these concepts, but how can you really apply them to your own life?

This is what the chapter on implementation is all about, and it helps you plan a lifelong change in your health focus to live these principles and truly experience long term health, greater happiness, and extended longevity.

For five years I amended and improved these materials which now include a lot more information and helpful concepts for students wanting to improve their longevity and those of others.

I transcribed my videos and other materials to this book so you can read it all, and later hear it in an AudioBook.

This book is priced pretty inexpensively, compared to the online training and certification program which sells in total for $1,995 USD. If you are interested in taking the entire online program at a major discount, then please contact me at:

Marty@personal-longevity.com

Hope you enjoy these materials since when applied correctly they will significantly change your life.

PLP Concepts Overview

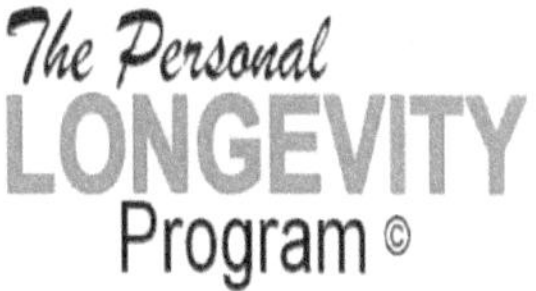

(Transcription of overview video)

Hello I'm Martin Ettington and I'd like to introduce you to the Personal Longevity Program which is an integrated holistic approach to long-term health. In this video we will only cover the high level concepts which comprise individual courses in the coaching certificate program for personal longevity.

The first concept is that long lived people exist and have existed for hundreds of thousands of years. We cover in the first course all about their records; along with people not only in places you might think like India, but in Europe and the United States-people who've lived long lives and well documented cases.

We discuss people who have lived well over the age of 120 and even the case of a Chinaman who lived to 256 years old. Plus a lot of mythology about people who have lived even longer lives so you get an idea that extending your life much longer than we think is currently medically and scientifically possible is certainly something that can happen.

The second course's concept has to do with finding your souls purpose. The point of wanting to live a long life is to know what your purpose in life is, so we go through some readings and some exercises to help you determine where soul's purpose in life is. Then doing goals as a fundamental concept so you will know the motivations in your life.

Third is the "Psychology of Living" also known by certain practitioners as "Removing the death Urge". The psychology of living has to do with seeking a positive image about your ability to live a long time. We tend to be programmed from birth about the idea that we are going to go through certain stages in our life as a child, as a teenager, and as adults. It's about reprogramming your subconscious as to the possibilities of a long life.

I've also learned in my life that it is very important to be able open your heart to unconditional love. When you're able to love unconditionally it also helps increase the strength of your immune system and fight off disease. So this is an aspect of spiritual growth. The courses also cover unconditional love and energy body forces. Managing your energy body is an important component of who you are in having energy working properly in your body and is another aspect of health for the length of longevity.

There are many types of scientific and medical research which are being done today and which will contribute to human longevity in the future.

Do you know that the average lifespan in the United States in 1900 was only about 40 years? We have doubled lifespan in the last century with current technologies but things under way in terms of scientific and medical improvements will help extend your lives further.

Also in this course on longevity we will cover a lot of the concepts which are being researched by scientists today. There are suggestions for more things you can do to do to use this science to improve your health along with physical supplements.

A unique thing that I thought about and decided to offer in these courses has to do with all my experiences in prophecy and how I was able to change outcomes on accidents that would occur to me by using simple exercises you can learn to change these outcomes. If you're in great health often the biggest thing you have to worry about are accidents.

We also provide guidelines you can follow on a daily basis and plans you can make to live healthier and happier and have a much longer life than you ever thought possible.

Thank you for listening !

Book 1 Video Introduction

(Video Transcription Follows)

Hello I'm Marty Ettington and I'd like to welcome you to this class number one on the Personal Longevity Program.

The subjects we are going to cover in this course happen to be records of long lived people, and mythical records of people who we can't document who had very long possible lives in the three bodies we all have. Spiritual, Energy, and Physical bodies and a synchronization which helps produce longevity in us.

Back in 2008 I was interested in a subject to write about and I'd always read that Yogis in India might live hundreds of years, so I decided to research that. So I'm looking at those records I found out that not only people in India, but in Europe, the U.S., and all over the world live and have lived to ages well beyond 150 and more. I must have found the records of a hundred people that lived to ages that Medical Sciences doesn't consider possible.

For example there is Li-Ching-Yung who had an article about himself in the New York Times about 1933 who lived to 256 years.

Even longer claimed lives of people who we might call mythical because we just don't have the documentation, and include people like Abdel Aziz El Habachi who was supposedly 674 years when he died in 1863 in Cairo. Supposedly he was there for the founding of Cairo too.

Or what about the Bible and the ages there which are outrageous that are claimed. There was Methuselah who was supposed to live 969 years old. Well we don't have any documentation to tell for sure.

We are going to cover some high level concepts also. The reality of the spirit that is the core of our being that lives in a timeless and space less realm. And the analogies of how black holes and big bang through science show that maybe that is the realm that existed.

A process I call synchronization. Synchronization of our three bodies which helps bring long-term health down into our physical being. And how the process that we call Enlightenment and Immortality are related. That the Enlightenment that you go through-the connection with your spirit is a critical component of longevity.

And we will look at Longevity Myths. Extremely long lived people that are living hundreds or thousands of years. That are not really documented but are something that's been reported by many people.

Also there are additional resources in this course. I put a few extra books on immortality in resources section
There are presentations and documents on all the people who are mythical immortals and additional resource links to other books and documents you can purchase or download information on longevity and immortality.

Don't forget to take your course test if you are going to be working on your certificate for the PLP. Good luck on the course and thank you very much.

Video of Long Lived Persons

(Long Lived Persons News Reports-Video Compilation-Transcription Follows)

This 120 year Indian woman is refusing to age. How does she do it? She says "eating well comes first and foremost". Somalakka is alive and well in the southern state of Tamil Nadu. Her daily routine is fairly normal. Save for the wrinkles and the bend in her back that give away her age—she is as fit as her granddaughters for all practical purposes. Living alone, she gets up early in the morning and does all of the household chores; from sweeping to cleaning and cooking -all on her own. Her favorite pastimes are reading newspapers, watching television, and going to a store in the village. "I have not gotten sick so far-I used to eat traditional foods such as cali, wheat, and maize. And I never ate any kind of fast food. Nowadays people love such food and fall sick, but I don't like to eat any such fast food. Amrawathy her granddaughter says "Our grandmother is the eldest among all of her brothers and sisters. Six other siblings died and now only four of her sisters are alive-including our grandma who is now 120 years old-and her other sisters are 110 years old. She now has more than 70 grandchildren." It seems that anyone can live the way the Somalakka does--but can everyone live to 120? That is something that only time will tell.

When he was born the world was a different place, and that's not surprising since it was the 19th century. Artize went to meet the man who claims to be the oldest person on the planet. The October revolution, the Russian Revolution, even the birth and death of two world wars. This man has seen them all because he claims to be 121 years old. Magonya Yazotof says he is the oldest person living in Russia and perhaps across the globe. People come to visit and talk to him and today Magonya has agreed to share some of his secrets to a long life with us too. Despite only humble surroundings Magonya says his neighborhood has provided him with the elixir of life. "I eat only what I raise myself. I drink milk and eat milk products and vegetables from my garden. All my life I was a farmer. I worked a lot with buffalos and horses. Hard work is good for you. While his body may not be as nimble as it once was, his soul remains strong and determined. All his life he strictly followed old religious traditions. He prays five times per day and does all the preparations himself. The official information we could find about Magonya dates back to the 1960s when he moved to Dagestan. In these documents it is said he was born in 1890 and there is also a database about him and his family. However, the rest of the archive to prove his life was destroyed in a fire in the 1930s in Chechnya where he was born.

A 150 year old man in Bangladesh. (Video showing and old man's home and village—sound track is in Tamil) Haji Khdem Hossain Sikhdar. Haji is 150 years old. Video shows him washing and putting on a shirt. He uses a magnifying glass to read. He was born in 7/2/1860. He is wearing a skullcap, has a white beard and is talking with a reporter. He was still alive as of 4/1/2013 and walking around with a cane. He lives in Madaripur, Bangladesh. He looks quite healthy. Showing records of him in an old school almanac.

A video of Shirali Mislimov who lived to 168 years old. Meet Shirali Mislimov—probably the world's oldest man. This mountain villager claims to be 163, and he credits hard work and a simple life for his longevity. The Caspian Sea region has dozens of centenarians. Shirali believes that the surrounding mountains are so high that the Angel of Death cannot reach him. A tea totalar and tobacco abstainer, Shirali's advice is a simple and direct philosophy. He says that families, neighbors , and nations should be good to each other. Wisdom of the Ages.

(Narrator talking in Hindu) New video on Devraha Baba who lived to 250 years. See video of a hunched over man who is walking to the left to a raised wooden structure which is his home. He was known as the "Ageless Yogi". He was known as a sadhu who preached harmony between religious communities. Video showing him lecturing to his devotees saying a prayer with them.

Physical Immortality Book Chapter 5

(An Extract from the book: "Physical Immortality: A History and How to Guide")

Considering the skepticism with which most people view records of very long lifetimes, I thought it would be useful to compile a list of as many long lived persons as possible; to show that these records exist and people really have lived lives of extraordinary length.

Nothing will convince somebody who has a closed mind or has to see the person's making these claims themselves. However, this list may start most people questioning that what they have been told all their lives about the limits to living; which are completely wrong.

Most of the persons listed were either from Europe, or North and South America.
I think the reason for this is that records have been better kept in the West in recent centuries. There were most probably as many persons living in Africa and Asia who lived long lives—we just don't have their records.

Also included in this chapter is a section on physical immortals to show that the possible length of physical life may be much longer than any of us can imagine; I.E. 9,000 years.

Below is a list from several sources which can be verified by going to the original records.

a.   Records of numerous long lived individuals

Ages 120-129

The oldest age that the Guinness Book of World Records recognizes is Jeanne Louise Calment (Born 21 February

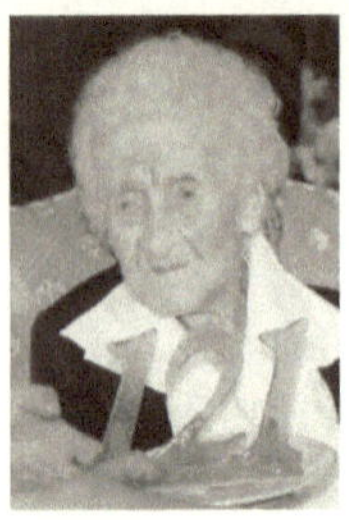

1875 – 4 August 1997, 10:45 CET). She had the longest confirmed human life span in history, living 122 years and 164 days (44,724 days total). She lived in Arles, France, for her entire life, and outlived both her daughter and grandson.

From the Immortality Article:

Eglebert Hoff was a lad driving a team in Norway when the news was brought that Charles I was beheaded. He died in Fishkill, N.Y., in 1764 at the age of one hundred and twenty-eight. He never used spectacles, read fluently, and his memory and senses were retained until his death, which was due to an accident.

Ages 140-149

Among the Mission Indians of Southern California there are reported instances of longevity ranging from one hundred and twenty to one hundred and forty.

Lieutenant Gibbons found in a village in Peru one hundred inhabitants who were past the century mark, and another credible explorer in the same territory records a case of longevity of one hundred and forty. This man was very temperate and always ate his food cold, partaking of meat only in the middle of the day.

Ages 150-159

In the chancel of the Honigton Church, Wiltshire, is a black marble monument to the memory of G. Stanley, a gentleman, who died in 1719, aged one hundred and fifty-one.

And in Acsadi & Nemeskeri, p.17 & Toronto Evening Telegram, 9 Sept., 1939; 26 April, 1942. (Also in the Longevity Article (7))

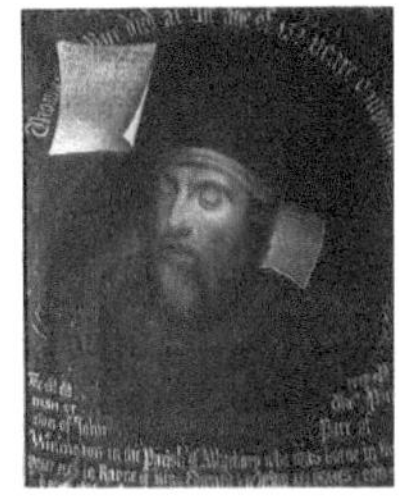

Thomas Parr, 152, died 1635, in England. Thomas Parr (or Parre), among Englishmen known as "old Parr," was a poor farmer's servant, born in 1483. He remained single until eighty. His first wife lived thirty-two years, and eight years after her death, at the age of one hundred and twenty, he married again. Until his one hundred and thirtieth year he performed his ordinary duties, and at this age was even accustomed to thresh.

He was visited by Thomas, Earl of Arundel and Surrey, and was persuaded to visit the King in London. His intelligence and venerable demeanor impressed everyone, and crowds thronged to see him and pay homage. The journey to London, together with the excitement and change in mode of living, undoubtedly hastened his death, which occurred in less than a year. He was one hundred and fifty-two years and nine months old, and had lived under nine Kings of England. Harvey examined his body and at the necropsy his internal organs were found in a most perfect state. His cartilages were not even ossified, as is the case generally with the very aged. The slightest cause of death could not be discovered, and the general impression was that he died from being over-fed and too-well treated in London. His great-grandson was said to have died in this century in Cork at the age of one hundred and three. Parr is celebrated by a monument reared to his memory in Westminster Abbey.

Of course who could forget Shirali Mislimov! There are many references to Shirali Mislimov including the January 1972 issue of National Geographic. However from Toronto Evening Telegram, 20 May, 1971 & the Ottawa Citizen, 13 Feb., 1967, p.18 & Life, 16 Sept.,1966, p.121 & Gris & Merlin, p.88-115 & Time, 17 Sept., 1973 we have this:

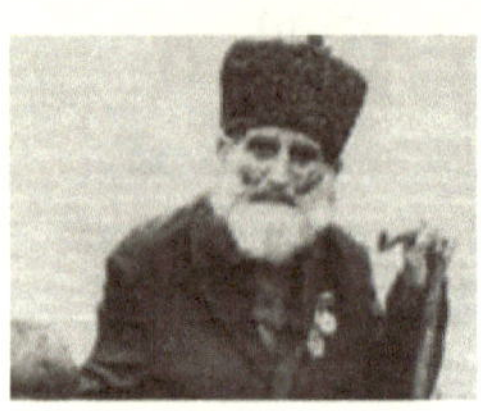

Shirali Mislimov, 168, Died 1973, in Azerbaijan, USSR.
On his birthday (1971) he rose at dawn to do his daily chores in the garden and orchard. Among his well-wishers were doctors who gave him his annual physical and judged his health perfect. He has never been ill, though forced to give up riding horseback recently.

At 160 he journeyed to the capital city (his first visit). There a doctor recorded his pulse at 72 and blood pressure at 120/75, and this was after a three story climb! He neither smoked or drank. Survived by his third wife, 107 years old, 219 other family members, including a grandchild aged 100 years.

b.   LI CHING-YUN: The Longest Lived person of record-256 Years

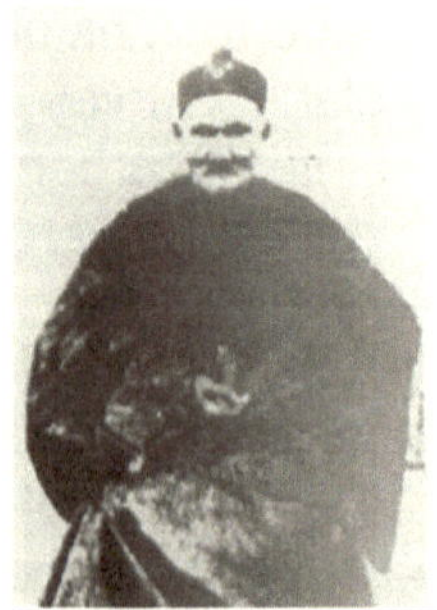

Below is an excerpt of an article from the New York Times (10):

<u>The New York Times, Saturday, May 6, 1933</u>

LI CHING-YUN DEAD; GAVE HIS AGE AS 197

"Keep Quiet heart, Sit Like a Tortoise, Sleep Like a Dog,"
His advice for a Long Life. Inquiry Put Age At 256.
He was reported to have buried 23 wives and had 180
descendants – sold herbs for first 100 years.

Peiping, May 5 – Li Ching-Yun, a resident of Kaihsien, in
the Province of Szechwan, who contended that he was
one of the world's oldest men and said he was born in
1736 – which would make him 197 years old – died today.

A Chinese dispatch from Chungking telling of Mr. Li's
death said he attributed his longevity to peace of mind and
that it was his belief every one could live at least a century
by attaining inward calm.

Compared with estimates of Li Ching-Yun's age in
previous reports from China, the above dispatch is
conservative. In 1930 it was said Professor Wu Chung-
Chien, dean of the department of Education in Minkuo
University, had found records showing Li was born in 1677
and that Imperial Chinese Government congratulated him
on his 150th and 200th birthdays.
A correspondent of The New York Times wrote in 1928
that many of the oldest men in Li's neighborhood asserted
their grandfathers knew him as boys and that he was then
a grown man.

According to the generally accepted tales told in his
province. Li was able to read and write as a child, and by
his tenth birthday had traveled in Kansu, Shansi, Tibet,
Annam, Siam and Manchuria gathering herbs. For the first

hundred years he continued at this occupation. Then he switched to selling herbs gathered by others.

Wu Pei-Fu, the warlord, took Li into his house to learn the secret of living to 250. Another pupil said Li told him to "keep a quiet heart, sit like a tortoise, walk sprightly like a pigeon and sleep like a dog."

According to one version of Li's married life he had buried away twenty-three wives and was living with his twenty-fourth, a woman of '60.' Another account, which in 1928 credited him with 180 living descendants, comprising eleven generations, recorded only fourteen marriages. This second authority said his eyesight was good; also, that the finger nails of his right hand were very long, and "long" for a Chinese might mean longer than any finger nails ever dreamed of in the United States.

One statement of The Times correspondent which probably caused skeptical readers to believe Li was born more recently that 1677, was that "many who have seen him recently declare that his facial appearance is no different from that of persons two centuries his junior."

An article from the May 15, 1933 issue of Time magazine titled:

Tortoise-Pigeon-Dog

In the province of Szechwan in China lived until last week Li Ching-Yun. ... By his own story he was born in 1736, had lived 197 years. By the time he was ten years old he had traveled in Kansu, Shansi, Tibet, Annam, Siam and Manchuria gathering herbs. ... Some said he had buried 23 wives, was living with his 24th-a woman of 60, and had descendants of eleven generations. The fingernails of his

venerable right hand were six inches long. Yet to skeptical Western eyes he looked much like any Chinese 60-year-old. In 1930 Professor Wu Chung-Chieh, dean of the department of education at Chengtu University, found records that the Imperial Chinese Government had congratulated one Li Ching-Yun in 1827 on his birthday. The birthday was his 150th, making the man who died last week—if it was the same Li Ching-Yun, and respectful Chinese preferred to think so—a 256-year-old.
More about Li Chang Yun from the *Toronto Evening Telegram,* 26 April, 1942:

LI CHING-YUN, 256, died May, 1933, Szechuan Province, China.

At the age of 100 he was awarded by the Chinese Government a special Honor Citation for extraordinary services to his country. This document is available in existing archives. It is reported that he gave a series of 28 lectures at the University of Sinkiang when he was over 200 years old. He attributed his longevity to his life-long vegetarian diet and regular use of rejuvenating herbs plus "inward calm".

 A renowned herbalist, he used Fo-Ti-Tieng and ginseng daily in the form of tea. He enjoyed excellent health, outlived 23 wives, and kept his own natural teeth and hair. Those who saw him at age of 200 testified that he did not appear much older than a man in his fifties.

A researched Li Chang(Ching) Yun is featured in this 1980 book: "The Seed of the Woman" by Arthur C. Custance

Li Ching Yun is also featured in the recent book: "Qigong Teachings of a Taoist Immortal: The Eight Essential Exercises of Master Li Ching-Yun" by Stuart Alve Olson

Enlightenment and Spirituality

(From the book "Enlightenment and Immortality")

The Ego In Our Lives

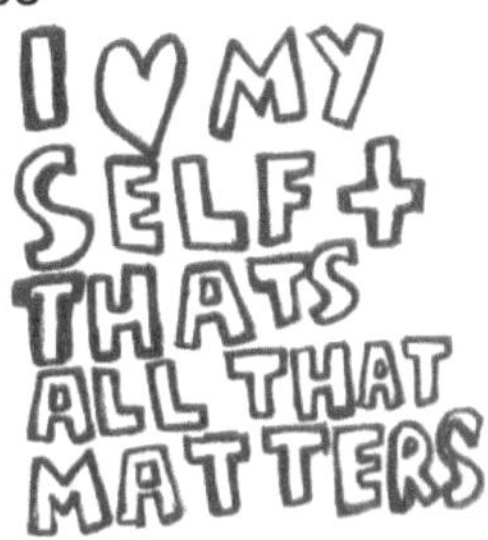

I was given a great gift before the beginning of my life, and I've only recently realized how great that gift was.

This gift was me being blessed with a continuous memory from before my conception--through birth—and until now.

I have clear experiences of remembering before my birth: Breaking off from a larger consciousness, choosing my mother, being in her womb, birth, and as a young baby.

Here is what I learned from remembering the incarnation and birth process….

The core of our being-our eternal spirit- tries to bring itself forward into our lives in each new incarnation.

We are all born with a piece of the spirit in us as the core of our consciousness.

As a newborn babe our minds are almost all made up of that spirit-and a sense of perception and curiosity about the world.

As the baby consciousness grows we learn about the world. While we do this we acquire an Ego. This Ego is part of our growth and helps us discern how to live in the world around us successfully.

It is a natural part of the growth of a baby to build this shell of thoughts and emotions around their spirit to become more aware of how to live in the world. Without this discernment we can't relate to our parents or our surroundings.

An analogy of this process might be that after shellfish drop older shells which are too small, they are very soft and vulnerable until their skin hardens into a new shell.

The building of our Ego shell is a similar protective mechanism.

The simple fact of learning to cry to get our mother's attention is how we learn to communicate to satisfy the needs of our bodies and to build the connection with our Mom and Dad; who help nurture us spiritually, emotionally, and physically.

I remember being hungry in my crib as a newborn baby and the only way I had to communicate was to cry—which babies do very effectively.

The usefulness of my crying was reinforced every time I did it—because I was hungry, had pooped or peed, or just wanted attention. Also, when I was hot, cold, or just unhappy.

This process steadily builds the infant ego as we all come to believe that our crying and desires control the universe around us.

As we become more aware and able to communicate, we start to understand that we are interacting with other beings—our parents and our family.

When I was about two years old I was sitting on the floor of my parent's living room watching cartoons on television. All of a sudden I felt like I had wakened from a dream. I saw everything around me much more clearly, and knew that I was alive and living in the world. It was my "I think therefore I am" moment.

I interpret this experience as being the moment my Ego congealed into a solid part of my consciousness. Everything going on around me became more understandable and clearer.

Parents naturally start to cut back on the total infant service as the child grows because they want the child to do age appropriate work for itself—feeding itself, using a toilet, getting dressed—all the steps a child goes through when they grow.

This process continues as we go to school and grow into adulthood.

Many people feel an emptiness as they grow and want to know more about themselves and why they are on this earth—they are searching for a connection to their eternal spirit.

Unfortunately, it's not so easy because the whole process of our growth into adults is normally in an environment which continues to value us as egocentric beings.

Take sports, grades, and all forms of competition. These are not bad—they are just part of everyday life and we are taught to make all of these activities and corresponding goals part of who we are.

This process naturally leads to us being centered in our artificial egos and we value the events and processes of the world as the main reality which we understand.

When we start exploring about who we really are, it is a learning process. Many of us turn to the religions in the cultures we are raised in.

Many of us have more of a passion and want to answer questions like:

- Why are we here?
- Who or what is God?
- Is my religion the best or only path to understanding?
- What is the meaning of life?

For most people with other priorities in life it may seem that we will never have time to explore the meaning of our lives and reach through our Ego to rebuild a deep connection with our spirit.

The growth of the Ego in each of us is a natural part of our lives on earth. However, we each have to make a conscious decision if we want to learn to feel the connection with our eternal spirit.

Longevity and Spirituality

I believe that our purpose in life is to experience this earth and evolve on it as spiritual beings.

A fortunate few learn how to feel the presence of the spirit in our everyday lives. Those persons become more and more enlightened as they build this connection with their spirit. It may be through learning prayer in a traditional religion like Christian Catholicism, or through meditation from the eastern philosophies and religious teachings.

Most people become caught in the everyday illusions of life and live with unhappiness in many forms due to their illusions.

This is where the expected roles of aging in a society create limitations.

The natural sequence in all societies is to be born, grow into adulthood, work, marry, have children, raise the children, retire, live a few years, and then die.

It seems a terrible tragedy that most of the people ever born on this earth are so caught up in the travails of everyday life that they never get beyond the packaged beliefs they are raised in to see the truth of their spirit for themselves.

Most people's free time for self-examination is very limited due to the daily activities of their lives—even into old age. We are talking about 99% of the population.

What can be done about this problem? How are we to help the masses have the opportunity for spiritual growth and self-fulfillment into becoming more realized beings?

After much thought and meditation I've concluded that helping each of us to have the potential for much longer lives than is now common would help us address what I would like to call the "life gap of enlightenment".

In my separate research and writings I've documented many persons who have lived well over the age of 150 years—some into the several hundred year range.

I now believe that my interest in the subject some years ago was driven by a subconscious spiritual knowledge of the importance extended longevity to create more opportunities for our spiritual growth.

Think about it—adding many more years beyond the normal lifetime naturally provides a greater opportunity for an individual's introspection and growth.

Once a person reaches the age of a "Senior" (commonly starting the in the fifties and beyond), they have experienced most of what normal life has to offer—love, careers, family, death of those close to you, accomplishment, and the seeing the results of their efforts here on earth. What is left?

The older one gets, the more they have "boredom" with the world and want to learn about their reason for being. This curiosity may come out of hiding in their subconscious after a lifetime of being suppressed below the other priorities of living in the world day to day.

Providing more time for a person to search for the truth in their lives thus allows them to have a greater chance to reach a greater enlightenment about themselves and a greater connection with their spirit.

It's also interesting to note that when studying the lives and teachings of very old persons—these people know that one of the main components of extreme longevity is being centered in the spirit.

I use as an example the well documented case of Li-Ching-Yung who lived to 256 years and who said his secret to a long life was:

"Keep Quiet heart, Sit like a Tortoise, Sleep like a Dog"

A "quiet heart" in the speech of the east refers to being in touch with your core being or spirit. Sitting like a tortoise also has to do with living in a slower and more thoughtful way.

So we can see that living with a closer connection to our spirit is not only a way to reach a more enlightened and happier state within us, but the action of doing that brings that spirit down into our bodies to increase our overall health and longevity.

Now we have a connection between extended longevity and the spiritual value of that additional lifespan.

One could say that the search for the spiritual connection in our lives also has a byproduct of extending our lives.

To what end do we want to do this? My intuition tells me that the purpose is to allow many more of us to become realized beings in this life.

Isn't that what the cycle of birth and death is all about? To become a further evolved and realized being at the end?

To become more spiritually evolved is to become more enlightened. What is enlightenment? Do we understand what the state is that we are striving to reach?

More about Enlightenment

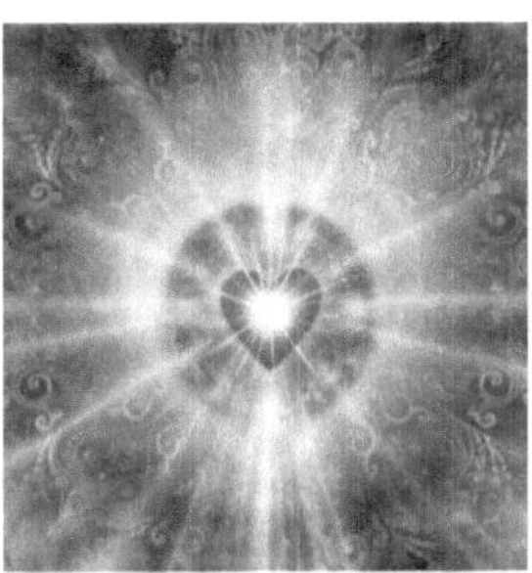

Enlightenment is a state that is impossible to understand unless you actually reach it.

Enlightenment is like a man who can see brilliant color in the land of the blind who only understand black and white.

<u>How is this state related to longevity and Immortality?</u>
- The more Enlightened you are, the easier it is to synchronize your Spirit, Energy, and Physical bodies (which we will discuss more later in this book)
- Enlightenment helps you to pierce the illusions most of us live under about ourselves and our environment—and our illusions about death
- Happiness allows you to have more positive outlook on life and to visualize positively about your health and future
- Many immortals are enlightened, and the same is true of enlightened masters—most are as immortal as they choose to become
- The two concepts are directly related and balance each other
    - An immortal has much more time to perfect their enlightenment
    - An enlightened person has a much easier time perfecting their body to be immortal

<u>What is Enlightenment?</u>

Start by looking at what Enlightenment is not:
- Enlightenment is not getting something whether that's getting more knowledge or becoming spiritually advanced.
- We need to let go of what we think it means to be spiritual
- Enlightenment has nothing to do with living up to a spiritual ideals
- We need to let go of any preconceived ideas about what meditation practice is and what it will do for you.

One of my favorite sayings on enlightenment is from Andrew Cohen's book "Enlightenment is a Secret"
On Page 60: "*Spiritual is the very nature of what you already are. There is nothing to do about it except to realize it. Once you have made this discovery it's all over.*"

- Enlightenment is the continuous state of knowing that you are the source energy at all times in every moment of life.
- Enlightenment is something you are, not something you go and get. This is why enlightenment does not need to be sought.

Enlightenment cannot be discerned by reading about it, it can only be experienced
(Be Here Now-Baba Ram Dass)

First a foremost you must understand that you are a Spiritual being having a human experience.
You are the energy you a looking for.
Right here. Right NOW.

This practice is simply an exploration of what is already present in you.

Enlightenment is a certainty that never leaves you. (Master Nasargadata)

It is a certainty that is so profound it can be called "remembering," because the truth of your being is so constant it becomes impossible to forget.
Certainty is more than the lack of doubt, fear and indecision.

Certainty is accompanied by trust.
When I look inside and see that I am nothing, that is wisdom, when I look outside, and see that I am everything, That's LOVE, and between these two my life turns.

Examples of the State of Enlightenment:
"Be Here Now" By Baba Ram Dass—Living in the Now
Feeling the Oneness of everyone and everything around you which is a state of boundless love
(Imagine feeling towards everyone and everything the way you feel about the person you love most in life)

Enlightenment in Opening the Heart
The gradual unfolding of our spirit within our bodies involves the opening of different chakras including the heart chakra.
The heart chakra is the center of love in our bodies and thus is our strongest connection to the spirit of God we can feel.
While I learned to open my crown chakra to take in vital forces energy and have a better connection to the divine at a young age, I didn't know what I was missing in my heart until very recently.

Learning exercises to open the heart chakra a couple of years ago gave me some very powerful but limited experiences with experiencing the energy of an unconditional love of God force within me.

This state is where you start to radiate Love to all of those around you and it fills your heart with happiness as you connect more broadly throughout your body and to others.

Recently my heart chakra opened completely on a daily basis and its (Ettington M. K., Love From The Heart, 2012) effect on me has been profound.
I love to sit for hours and just enjoy the heat and joy within my chest and my connection to everyone-it is like a drugged natural high.

I see all of my friends in a new light. This experience makes me realize that for most of my life I had a deep gap and loneliness in my heart which has only now been filled after living fifty plus years in this life. I had thought that intimacy with woman could fill that hole within me. That is not how it works.

Now, I realize the fallacy of that belief. We can really only fill loneliness with a connection to the spirit of God through our hearts.

This love from God is something I want to share with everyone and help everyone learn to open their hearts too.

The Limits of Enlightenment
Unlike many other seekers I believe that enlightenment is a continuous process—not a single blaze of light and understanding.

We live in an infinite Universe and there are beings of much greater power and glory than we can conceive. Every time we reach a new state of enlightenment we find that the road ahead is still infinitely long and forever full of wonderful mysteries.

Why not take advantage of living our lives as fully and as long as possible to evolve to our full potentials?

The Importance of Extended Longevity

For a few people, spiritual awakenings come early in life because of positive karma, or through a spontaneous experience. However, most of us have to work at it for many years to make breakthroughs.

Even though I have been a spiritual seeker most of my life, my awakenings have been gradual over a long period of time; and are still going on.

In the nineteen sixties when I was a boy there wasn't much aside from the Bible at our house in small town in upstate New York as a guide for the spiritual path. Don't get me wrong-the Bible is a great document of History, Religion, and Spirituality—but there is much more to learn in other texts and experiences about spiritual paths.

I did read a book called "Stranger Than Science" By Frank Edwards which had a series of unbelievable and supposedly true stories which posed some major questions to me that nobody I knew could answer.

At the RPI where I was studying engineering in the early seventies I found a mentor—a physics graduate student in his forties named Sam-who was also an accomplished clairvoyant and healer.

Sam introduced me to meditation and the opening of my crown chakra. This was a major milestone in my life and the results were incredible.

As my vital forces increased and I opened up spiritually and psychically.

I had experiences of prophecy, astral projection, learned to do healing, and many other awakenings. I was only nineteen years old.

For the next several decades my career, family, and the routines of daily life became my priorities and although I meditated and continued to read a lot I felt stuck –that I was not spiritually advancing.

My next milestone was aided with technology- when I bought a new type of Meditation CD (from Centerpointe) which played two different frequency tones in my ears and turned my haphazard meditations into consistently deep and steady ones.

Over a period of eight of nine years, I continued to become calmer and more centered. That period was also when I had many prophecies about major events and my life.

(Profiled in my book Prophecy: A History and How to Guide)

Then I seemed to plateau again for several years….

My divorce started in 2008 and this led me to write my well known book on Immortality: "Physical Immortality: A History and How to Guide"

The other effect of my divorce was to lead me to re-evaluate my life—my goals, my social life, and what I wanted to do for the rest of my life.

I took up new practices including learning Reiki Healing— where I went to numerous classes and took several levels of training and certification.

This process included more exercises to open chakras and manipulate vital forces.

Then I learned a exercise to open the heart chakra which resulted in a couple of amazing experiences of powerful unconditional love.—which each lasted a few hours then want away again.

Two years and many spiritual groups and classes later my heart chakra opened fully and brought me to a whole new level of awareness.

My heart opening has become a great blessing in my life and is even more powerful than my crown chakra opening several decades ago.

To feel the love of God in my heart fills a hole that I know now I've had my whole life—and I didn't even realize how empty my heart was.

To feel filled with love and this life force pulsing throughout my chest is a wonderful experience.

It is hard to explain the joy of feeling a connection of love to everyone and everything around one-but it is worth it.

I know now that as my life goes on I will continue to develop spiritually and will have many more wonderful experiences.

So far my spiritual journey has been about forty-five years, and I'm still having major experiences as time goes on.

These continued experiences give me a strong desire to want to stay on this earth as long as I can-to build an ever deeper connection to my spirit.

I'm just getting to what most people would call "Senior" adult status, but my spiritual growth is constantly renewing itself and will continue to do so for many more years.

Having another couple of centuries or more in my life will not be enough time to explore and experience everything I want to in this varied and beautiful world we live on.

Extended Longevity provides the additional time most of us need to learn and experience meaning and spiritual growth in our lives.

Synchronization of Spirit, Energy, Physical Body

You are not just your physical body. Your being includes a Spiritual Core, an Energy Body, and Physical Body.

These are concepts which are woven into many religions and philosophies, with related energy body concepts mostly being understood in the East more than the West.

Many believe that your entire being consists of at least three states as described below.

<u>The Spirit</u>

Here we mean the spirit which is your "soul" or core of your being. An individual's spirit is one with the God spirit and is present in every person and every being. It exists outside of time and space. This is a place some call "no time and no space". It is everywhere present simultaneously.

The spirit exists in all things and each person has that same core spirit within them.

We can learn to live focused more in the spirit through a variety of religious, meditational, and philosophical traditions.

The Energy Body

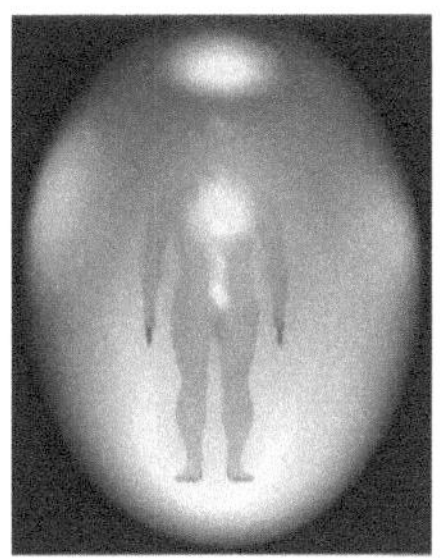

Some organizations like the Hindus and Theosophists believe we have multiple energy body levels. The Theosophists believe there are at least six distinct energy bodies.

Many other traditions only talk about one energy body which provides the life force to energize our physical bodies.

The acupuncture meridians and chakras are all parts of the energy body which exists in very close proximity to the physical body.

The aura is also a manifestation of the energy body too, which overlaps your physical body.

Many people claim to be able to see "auras" including this Author. The aura is the physical energy manifestation of the energy body. All living people have an aura and one can tell a lot about their health by how their aura looks.

The Physical Body

This is the body most of us know, and that most of us think is all of us that exists. This is the body we want to heal and energize to achieve physical immortality.

Exercises done on the physical body also affect the energy body.

Herbal supplements work from the physical body to help correct energy flows in your energy body.

How the Bodies Work Together

Spiritual development exercises and physical exercises help increase the synchronization of these bodies.

By bringing the absolute peace and stillness of the spirit down into the energy and physical bodies you increase the perfection and health of those bodies.

This is since in the normal course of events the stresses of our life cause more randomness or entropy in our energy and physical bodies. These stresses of daily life age us prematurely and cause disease.

We can repair our energy and physical bodies by integrating them better with the spiritual body; and getting the energies to flow in the correct patterns, chakras, and meridians, and with more vital force.

The specific practices to extend your longevity are provided in much more detail in "Physical Immortality: A History and How to Guide".

Synchronization is a holistic approach of working on our entire being to help us become healthier, happier, and to have much more profound life experiences.

Connecting to the Spirit

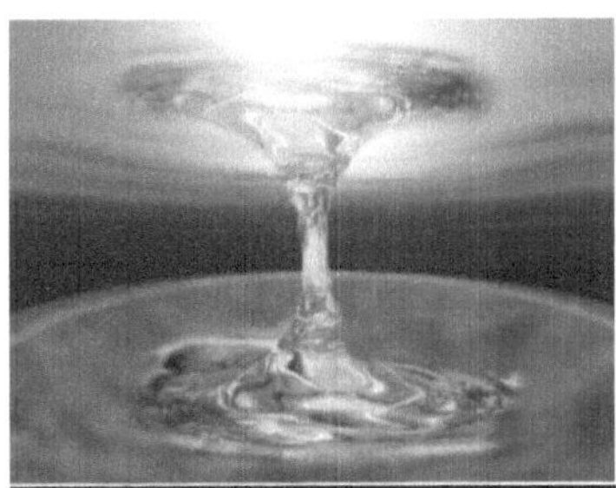

The Importance of Stillness

How does spiritual growth help one stay healthy; and what is stillness?

The ideas I'm going to discuss here relate to eastern Asian concepts of the spirit as taught mainly in China and India.

Buddhism, Taoism, Zen, and other eastern religions and philosophies all teach that the spirit is the core of our being; and that our physical bodies are just an extension of that spirit into the physical level of existence.

By learning to let your mind or ego release its hold on the illusion of our current existence, we become aware of the spirit behind or at the core of our being. This spirit is the pure oneness of God and exists in no time and no space. (A concept which we really can't envision with our minds or egos only).

There are many techniques taught to get closer to realizing the core of a person's being. These techniques all involve practicing spiritual growth, love, and/or meditation with a goal of enlightenment.

There are thousands of books and practices on this subject so I will not try to duplicate them in this short synopsis.

The Chinese stress that the stillness and oneness obtained through spiritual growth are one of the main keys to keeping the body healthy for a long life. Many Taoist techniques and teachings stress the achievement of "stillness" as a prelude to physical immortality.

The stillness I'm referring to is found mainly through meditation. In Christian terms it is often referred to as the "Peace that passes all understanding".

It is hard to describe the feeling of stillness since it is like when you first wake up in the morning after a deep sleep—but even quieter and deeper.

The feeling of stillness has a strong effect on your body—it seems to make the randomness of your cells quiet down into a more restful state.

Meditation is taught many places; I've even found a company which sells CDs that help even beginners achieve deep states of relaxation that usually takes advanced Yogis years of practice.

Stillness is not something achieved overnight but takes years, (even with modern advanced CD techniques) to start showing results.

However, the effects of stillness practices probably have the most profound effects on your body's aging as anything else I can recommend.

This is since as you start to achieve stillness, your Ego is realizing its core is really part of the spirit—not a separate mind. The spirit exists outside time and space. This connection with your spirit has a profound health effect on the body in terms of peace and well-being.

When meditating in this state you can feel stillness penetrating your body.
It feels like your body is reaching a relaxed state never realized; even in sleep.
The state of the stillness of your spirit provides a modified blueprint for your body's health.

It is a lot of work to set aside time every day to meditate. The good news is you will find that after some weeks of practicing, this time becomes something you look forward to. This is since meditation is so relaxing it becomes a way to recharge you for daily activities in the world.

I also find that meditation makes my mind more alert when I wake up in the morning and gives me a sharper intellectual edge at work. If you are like me, you may sense strong danger if something bad will happen. All I can advise you is that if you do get a strong impression you should follow your intuition and take precautions to avoid that future situation.

Using the perceptions of our spirit to keep us safe is just making use of the abilities we all have. We can be as protected and safe as we desire.

Longevity through synchronization Video

(Video Transcription Follows)

I'd like to talk about a little bit about the theory of spiritual energy and physical body synchronization. As an engineer and technical person I always talk in terms of a hypothesis that you have to prove to yourself.

One way to prove it is that we will all have a reunion of all people that we teach and know in the year 2100 so you might want to mark that down on your calendar. The idea is that I think we probably all agree with is that we all have a core spirit which is part of the universal spirit and that the spirit exists outside of time and space.

We are going to talk about that a little more and the concepts of a timeless spirit that is a basis for all reality. And through thought it creates the energy body which then materializes the physical body. Therefore health and vitality depends on how well these three synchronize together. That's the basis of everything we are going to talk about this weekend.

That it's not any one specific practice but there are a lot of different things you can do which come from various sources which will all fit under this umbrella of how you can keep yourself young and vital.

Any questions about that?

We base this on many sources. A lot of historical experiences from thousands of people who have experienced enlightenment- who say that in that process- in that state of being-that the peace that they have internally helps stabilize their health and physical body.

There's a lot of exercises and we will cover a series of them talking about that approach. It's about personal experiences of being used outside of time and space.

And we will talk about spirit and the similarity or modern physics. And there's also a recent stories of quantum mechanics. Again, we are going to get into this later in the weekend to show you that there are actually some scientific analogies of the things we're talking about.

One example I will give you now is that-Does everyone know what an astronomical black hole is? -- If you heard that term? What a black hole is according to astrophysicists is a star that has a certain mass and size called a Swartzchild Radius-and if it is above that mass when it dies it will explode into a nova or supernova. If it's below that mass the star will collapse first into a dwarf, then a neutron star; then it will collapse into an infinitely small point. In that infinitely small point our knowledge of physics breaks down. All we can do is say that it must have gone to a point that is infinitely small where no time exists. And that what physicists understand about that.

So is that is that the same state that we talk about as a timeless and space-less state for our spirit? I think maybe it's a doorway into that.

We are going to talk about other analogies too, but I thought that would be the place to start.

In the energy body-let me just ask—Who has not seen the Chakra picture before? Anyone? OK Not to spend a lot of time on that except we are going through that in some of our exercises on energy meridians—So everybody's pretty familiar with the concept of the energy body and meridians? We're going to go into the different ways to manipulate that through meditation exercises.

In fact it's fair to say that most of what we are going to talk about this weekend and the reason we're starting with the first thing is a breath work exercise- is if you don't already know how to meditate or relax-it's something that is important to learn to follow our concepts and to follow our exercises.

So we're just going to do that to help everybody get on the same page as far as an approach and we can all use this weekend.

Different types of them are exercises like Tai-Chi or Kung Fu-Various types of Yoga-they all help to manipulate your energy.

We're going to do some exercises for instance where we talk about taking in energy through the crown and circulating around your body to various chakras.

And visualization techniques. Are all you pretty familiar with these techniques? Who is familiar with the concepts of visualization for affecting your future? - Almost everybody. We will do some visualization techniques. We are going to do the five Tibetan rights too.

So we believe the physical bodies are affected by the foods you eat. And that exercise provides a template to organize your body and as a vessel of your thoughts and energy to materialize into.

So again this is about Energy and Physical body Synchronicity.

Very long lived People

(Video Transcription Follows)

Now we'll get into some specific people and I've done a lot of searches both on the Internet, in books, and in various newspapers

And I'll mention that just recently I was doing a search on the New York Times database from 1852 to like 1960 and this was after I put all this together-I found another 20 plus people have lived over 130 years.

These are just records of people you won't find in the Guinness world book of records but people who did exist and are pretty well documented.

So the first one we are going to talk about is Catherine Fitzgerald Countess of Desmond who lived up until the year 1604 and she kind of looks pretty skeletal in this picture-this monograph. But she was alive and she walked every week to her local market town- a distance of 4-5 miles. Her teeth had started renewing before she died.

So she was pretty remarkable-and notice that that a lot of these very old people get regular daily exercise that a lot of us have quit doing. That's very important by itself. Forget all the studies about the importance of exercise. You can just see the effect from these old people.

Another one we will talk about is Dr. William Hotchkiss who reached the age of 140 years in 1895 and he was also a person who was probably involved mesmerism and claimed to treat people by magnetic process. Masonic records showed on it he was at least 121 years old.

Christian Jacobson Drakenberg-a very interesting history about this guy. He lived to 150 and he was a sailor for 91 years. Then he was captured by pirates and was a slave for 15 years. He got married at the age or 110. So he was known as the old man in the north and the stories are that even in old age he had tremendous strength and anybody who would shake his hand would feel like their hand was crushed because it was so strong.

According to some stories also when he died his body, mummified and didn't de-compose-and that's similar to other stories like Yogananda who had a very purified corpse. So there was something about his energy which helped keep his body very stable.

Thomas Parr 152 died in 1635. There is a link where you can download on a book on him. It was written in like 1632 or something before he died. It's really interesting reading this very old English about his life and the things he did and he performed ordinary servant duties until he was 130. So I guess they didn't have social security back then and he had to work pretty hard. He would visit the King in London; but what was really fascinating was the book was written about him in the time he lived. So that's pretty strong evidence that he really did live that long.

Robert Lynch a Negro slave. He recalled the great earthquake of 1692 and that the famous pirate Sir Henry Morgan who was also the last governor there. So he was probably 160 years old they said. Again somebody like that would not have had a birth certificate but the fact that he recalled these historical eras was some good evidence for what he was saying.

And we have Zero Aga. He was 164 years old when he died. And he came to the U.S. to visit. He worked as a porter for nearly 100 years and retired as a janitor.
So he was known as the world's oldest living man in the 1930s; and looks like he doesn't have a lot of energy- was around and was still kicking—he was a Kurd.

And then we have Javier Pereira- who was very well documented. In fact his country even made stamps about him-Columbia. And this is back in the 1950s-a 1956 stamp. He had remarkable feats of endurance, He could stand on one leg and pirouette. He could walk three blocks and climb stairs without losing his breath. He was known in his village as the old Indian who like to dance. He as fairly short too- only about 5 feet high. But he was a very long lifer of 169-so we are pushing up the age limit here.

Shirali Mislimov. Did anybody ever read articles about him in the National Geographic going back to the 1970s?- it had an article about him. So he's very well documented and he lived in Azerbaijan in an area where there's lots of people over one hundred. So he wasn't the oldest person who was very old but he was the oldest person who was documented. He had incredible blood pressure after a three story climb his pulse was 72 and blood pressure went 120/75. He was survived by his third wife and 219 other family members. A grandchild was over hundred years old. A very well documented case of 168.

Kentrigan-we only have this pictorial representation of him but the legend is that he founded on founded Glasgow Abbey in Scotland in the year 600 A.D. and lived to 185 And there is a story of his encounter with King Arthur's wizard Merlin. Not as well documented, but it is in the records of Glasgow Abbey.

Thomas Karn lived to 207 years. He lived through the reigns of numerous Kings of England. There is not a lot of information published about him but there were several different references to this guy's extreme longevity.

So now we are getting to the realm where people say "gee this is pretty weird-but is this for real?-- but we are going to go a little further.

The the best documented person we know about who lived a very long life was Li-Ching-Yung who lived up 256 years old and living in China. And he made these claims for his longevity. He was an herbalist for his first hundred years which may have had a big part to do with his longevity. He said "Keep a Quiet Heart, Sit like a Tortoise, and Sleep like a dog". He was very much into stillness practice.

Which is part of what we are going to talk about this weekend. Can we get older than that?

Well there are records of a guy named the Trailinga Swami A famed spiritual Yogi, who lived in India and he was reportedly about 300 years old when he decided to pass on. Again we don't have very solid records but we do have a picture of him. Notice he was even kind of fat--not that I recommend that—but he was able to stay healthy even being overweight.

This one I just threw in here because it's so fascinating. Imagine you are in the year 1876 if you talk to an official and claim you're at 615 years old and you have six wives all living. So they hauled him off to the insane asylum.

I just had to put this in here-it is not well documented— aside from the story.

How about a guy who was supposedly 674 years old. He was Abd el Aziz Habachi. This is from a book called Faras El Faras and supposedly he was even in the city of Cairo for its founding in 969 A.D. If that's true then he might have been over 900 years old when he died in 1859 A.D.

So that is the oldest person I've been able find so far that they claim was an actual historical person. What about people are still alive today?

Well, I found two news reports just the summer; one is a woman who's alive and discovered on her 130th birthday-there's a birthday cake there-living in the Soviet Republic of Georgia and she claims she was born July 8, 1880 and she is healthy and worked all her life-at home and on the farm. And she had a couple of Soviet era documents attesting this too. So this is a recent news from July 8 of this year.

Turinah is supposedly 157 years old and living in Sumatra. She has a very good memory, very clear hearing, and smoked the clove cigarettes. That would put her 35 years older Jeanne Calumet from the Guinness book world records.

So far we have gone through people that were supposed to be really historical people who lived a long time.

Common Threads-Lynn helped me compile this list is on these people all who had an interest in spending time in nature. In fact I've heard stories. One of the stories that Leonard Orr reports is a man who lived in Southeast Asia who was supposedly 400 years old. All he would do was every few months he would just go out and walk around in the woods for for 24 hours and kind of feel the life force-so that has something to do with longevity.

And they all had regular exercise-they all walked or hiked on a daily basis.

They spent lots of times with friends and relatives-so they had connections with people they weren't totally isolated.

And they enjoyed their work. If it stopped being enjoyable they would do something else.

And finally, a lot of them used different herbs. The two herbs that Li-Ching-Yung recommended for longevity-and easterners are another group in my book I talk about. These are the primary two- Ginseng and Fo-Ti-Tieng.

Those are very popular as longevity herbal supplements. Because he recommended them and some other persons who are very knowledgeable herbalists also do to.

Now we are going to talk about people that are reported to have lived a long time but for whom we have no other historical information.

We are going to push up the potential age limit a little more. So of course you all probably remember Genesis Chapter Five from the King James Version of the Bible. And does anybody see a pattern in these ages here? Because they go up to like 900 years and then they drop.

What might these ages have in relation to a major historical event that's report in the bible? Can anybody tell me? The Flood? Yes-because notice that the ages recorded were the highest before the flood and after the flood they dropped.

 A big factor in your longevity is a belief about death.

There's a guy named Ben Abba who used remote viewing to find a bunch of immortals around the world and he's published a blog and threatening to publish a book for a couple of yeas. He claims he found two persons-who I would put the suffix of immortal on who were 2800 years.

One agreed to talk to him-- and he had several interviews with him- he wrote the first chapter of this book which I've seen.

One of the things the guy told him is that he tries to get out every day and have lunch with somebody. He lives in a city around the Mediterranean. Of course this guy wouldn't be specific about which city. But he says that the person tries to get out every day and sit with somebody to maintain social contact. And we talk about that as a common thread among people. So I don't have a lot more information on this guy except Ben felt that the stories he had about the things he had done were credible.

How many of you have heard of Babaji as described in a number of books especially in Yogananda's book and also Lenard Orr who said he met him?

This I think is the highest potential length of life of anybody that we could find. A person supposed to be an ascended being. In other words he can materialize or dematerialize his body at will.

In fact one of the things I've read in different books because I'm interested in a lot of different spiritual or paranormal things is a book on Teleportation.

And one of things it said in this book is a learning these exercises- it was reported by different Yogi's is that you would be able practice Teleportation when you were in your 300s to 400s years old. So there may be certain abilities you learn as you spiritually develop.

That for most people will take much longer than a normal lifetime. I think of that because it would be something that you have to be quite old already to learn how to do-to dematerialize your body. He is kind of the endpoint to where we think a person might have lived to.

Longevity Myths

Persian Empire-The reigns of several shahs in the Shahnameh, an epic poem by Ferdowsi, are given as longer than a century:

• Zahhak, 1000 years.

• Jamshid, 700 years.

• Fereydun, 500 years.

• Askani, 200 years.

• Kay Kāvus, 150 years.

• Manuchehr, 120 years.

• Lohrasp, 120 years.

• Goshtasp, 120 years.

China Lucian wrote about the "Seres" (a Chinese people), claiming they lived for over 300 years.

• Zuo Ci who lived during the Three Kingdoms Period was said to have lived for 300 years.

• In Chinese legend, Peng Zu was believed to have lived for over 800 years during the Yin Dynasty (殷朝, 16th to 11th centuries BC).

• In traditional Daoism, the eight immortals are said to exist. Emperor Jimmu. Japan Some early emperors of Japan ruled for more than a century, according to the tradition documented in the Kojiki, viz., Emperor Jimmu and Emperor Kōan.

• Emperor Jimmu (traditionally, 13 February 711 BC – 11 March 585 BC) lived 126 years according to the Kojiki. These dates correspond to 126 years, 27 days, on the Julian and Gregorian calendars. However, the form of his posthumous name suggests that it was invented in the reign of Kammu (782–806), or possibly during the time in which legends about the origins of the Yamato dynasty were compiled into the Kojiki. Korea

• Taejo of Goguryeo (46/47 – 165) is generally accepted as having reigned in Korea for 93 years beginning at age 7. After his retirement, the Samguk Sagi and Samguk Yusa give his age at death as 118.

Roman empire In Roman times, Pliny wrote about longevity records from the census carried out in 74 AD under Vespasian.

In one region of Italy many people allegedly lived past 100; four were said to be 130, others even older.

The ancient Greek author Lucian is the presumed author of Macrobii (long-livers), a work devoted to longevity. Most of the examples Lucian gives are what would be regarded as normal long lifespans (80–100 years).

• Tiresias, the blind seer of Thebes, was alive for over 600 years (Lucian).

• Nestor lived over 300 years (Lucian).

• According to one tradition, Epimenides of Crete (7th, 6th centuries BC) lived nearly three hundred years.

Poland

• Piast Kołodziej, king of Poland, died in 861 legendarily age 120 (birth 740/741).

Czech Republic In legend, Praotec Čech ("forefather Czech", 342–680) lived 338 years.

And Přemysl, the Ploughman (founder of the Přemyslid dynasty) could have lived for more than 180 years (561–745).

Christianity

• Saint Servatius, bishop of Tongeren in continental Europe, died 13 May 384 according to consistent tradition. He was consecrated at the alleged age of 297, and is said to have lived for 375 years (birth 8/9 AD).

• Saint Shenouda the Archimandrite, a Coptic saint, lived c. 348–466 (117/118 years). He died on and is remembered on 7 Epip on the Coptic calendar (Sunday, 14 July, Julian).

• Welsh bard Llywarch Hen (Heroic Elegies) died c. 500 in the parish of Llanvor, traditionally about age 150.

• Saint Kevin of Glendalough died in 618, legendarily at age 120 (birth 497/498).

• Around 1912, the Maharishi of Kailas was said by missionary Sadhu Sundar Singh to be an over 300-year-old Christian hermit in a Himalayan mountain cave with whom he spent some time in deep fellowship. Singh said the Maharishi was born in Alexandria, Egypt, and baptized by the nephew of St. Francis Xavier.

• Scolastica Oliveri is said to have lived in Bivona, Italy, 1448–1578 (age 129/130), according to the archive of Monastero di San Paolo in Bivona located in Palermo.

Islam

• Abdul Azziz al-Hafeed al-Habashi (ال عزي زال ح ب شي ع ب د) (lived 581–1276 of the Hijra (11 June 1185 – 19 September 1859, 674 years, 100 days), i.e., 673/674 Gregorian years or 694/695 Islamic years, according to 19th-century scholars. Hinduism

• Devraha Baba (1477–1989) was rumored to be over 700 or even over 750 years old.

• Trailanga Swami reportedly lived in Kashi since 1737; the journal Prabuddha Bharata puts his birth around 1607 and his age 279 (almost 280), upon his death in 1887 on 26 December. His birth is also given as 1527 (age 359/360).

• The sadhaka Loknath Brahmacari reportedly lived 1730–1890 (age 159/160).

• Shivapuri Baba, also known as Swami Govindanath Bharati, was a Hindu saint who purportedly lived from 1826 to 1963, making him allegedly 137 years old at the time of his death. He had 18 audiences with Queen Victoria.

Buddhist saints

• LP Suwang (d.1995) was a holy Buddhist who entered Thailand in the 1920s. He was supposedly capable of miracles, and no one knew his exact age, not even his closest disciples. He died in 1995, at a claimed 200 years old, but rumored to be over 500 years old. The newest version claimed his birth as being in 1551, making him 444 years old. The subject of his age remains a mystery.

Falun Gong

• Chapter 2 of Falun Gong by Li Hongzhi (2001) states, "A person in Japan named Mitsu Taira lived to be 242 years old.

During the Tang Dynasty in our country, there was a monk called Hui Zhao [慧昭, 526–815] who lived to be 290 [288/289] years old.

According to the county annals of Yong Tai in Fujian Province, Chen Jun [陈俊] was born in the first year of Zhong He time (881 AD) under the reign of Emperor Xi Zong during the Tang Dynasty. He died in the Tai Ding time of the Yuan Dynasty (1325 AD), after living for 444 years." Theosophy/New Age

• Babaji is said to be an "Unascended Master" purportedly many centuries old who is claimed to live in the Himalayas. One of Babaji's disciples is said to be the Hindu guru Paramhansa Yogananda, who claimed to have met him. Many New Age people believe in the existence on the physical plane of this allegedly centuries old yoga master.

Political claims China

• A New York Times story announced the death on 5 May 1933 in Kaihsien, Szechwan, at the age of 197, of the Republic of China's Li Ching-Yuen (李青云, Li Qing Yun), who claimed to be born in 1736. A Time article noted that "respectful Chinese preferred to think" Li was 150 in 1827 (birth 1677), based on a government congratulatory message, and died at age 256.T'ai chi ch'uan master Da

Liu stated that Li learned qigong from a hermit over age 500.

United Kingdom

• The Shoreditch burial register for 28 January 1588 reads "Aged 207 years. Holywell Street. Thomas Carn" or "Carn", which supplied a traditional birth year of 1381. According to Old and New London, "the 2 should probably be 1".

Chapter 2 of Falun Gong by Li Hongzhi (2001) states, "According to records, there was a person in Britain named Femcath who lived for 207 years."

• Peter Torton reportedly died in 1724 age 185.

• A brief biography of Henry Jenkins, of Ellerton-on-Swale, Yorkshire, was written by Anne Saville in 1663 based on Jenkins's description, stating birth in 1501; he also claimed to recall the 1513 Battle of Flodden Field. However, Jenkins also testified in 1667, in favor of Charles Anthony in a court case against Calvert Smythson, that he was then only 157 or thereabouts. He was born in Bolton-on-Swale,and the date given, 17 May 1500, results in only a 1 year discrepancy with the age of 169 on his monument (he died 8 December 1670).

• A tombstone in Cachen churchyard near Cardiff, Glamorganshire, read, "Heare lieth the body of WILLIAM EDWARDS, of the Cairey, who departed this life the 24th of February, Anno Domini 1668, anno aetatis suae one hundred and sixty-eight".

• Joseph Surrington was reported as 160 (1637–1797). • The parish registers of Church Minshull, in the county of Chester, state, "1649 Thomas Damme of Leighton. Buried the 20th of February, being of the age of Seven-score and fourteen" (154 years), signed by vicar T. Holford and wardens T. Kennerly and John Warburton.

• A tombstone in Brislington, Bristol, reads, "1542 THOMAS NEWMAN AGED 153 This Stone was new faced in the Year 1771 to Perpetuate the Great Age of the Deceased."

• Mrs. Eckleston of Philipstown, King's-county, was stated to be 143 (1548–1691).

• Margaret Patten reportedly died in 1739 age 137.

United States of America Social Security:

• In the Social Security Death Index, the extreme age claim is of Anne Feinseth from New Jersey. She claimed to have been born February 12, 1809 and died February 24, 2004 at the alleged age of 195 years (ssn:135-42-7235).

• Elizabeth M. Mahony of California claimed birth on October 28, 1808, and died March 13, 2000 at the claimed age of 191 years, according to her death certificate.

• According to the July 20, 1876 New York Times, a man arrested in Newark, NJ named Colestein Veglin claimed to be 615 years old and to have 6 wives, all living. Following this proclamation, he was taken to an insane asylum for two days.

Hungary

• Netherlands envoy Hamelbraning reported in 1724 of the death in Rofrosh, Hungary, on January 5 of Peter Czartan, reportedly born 1539 and age 184.

Charles Hulbert, who reported Czartan's case in an 1825 collection, added that John (172) and his wife Sara (164) both died in Hungary in 1741 after 148 years of marriage. The Book "Validation of Exceptional Longevity" has the old couples last name as Rowin, while The Virgin Birth And The Incarnation puts John and Sara's married name as Rovin.

Pakistan

The 1973 National Geographic article on longevity also reported, as a very aged people, the Burusho or Hunza people in the Hunza Valley of the mountains of Pakistan.

Russia (Soviet Union)

Deaths officially reported in Russia in 1815 listed 1068 centenarians, including 246 supercentenarians (50 at age 120–155 and one even older). Time magazine considered that, by the Soviet Union, longevity had elevated to a state-supported "Methuselah cult".

The USSR insisted on its citizens' unrivaled longevity by claiming 592 people (224 male, 368 female) over age 120 in a 15 January 1959 census and 100 citizens of Russia alone ages 120 to 156 in March 1960. Such later claims were fostered by Georgian born Joseph Stalin's apparent hope that he would live long past 70.

Zhores A. Medvedev, who demonstrated that all 500-plus claims failed birth-record validation and other tests, said Stalin "liked the idea that [other] Georgians lived to be 100".

• An early 1812 Russian Petersburgh Gazette reports a man between ages 200 and 225 in the diocese of Ekaterinoslaw (now Dnipropetrovsk, Ukraine).

• Shirali Muslimov (26 March 1805? – 4 September 1973), of Barzavu, Azerbaijan, in the Caucasus mountains, was allegedly age 168 years, 162 days, based solely on a passport. National Geographic carried the claim.

The oldest woman in the USSR according to the Novosti Press Agency was supposed to have been Ashura Omarova from Daghestan, aged 195.

South Africa

• Emily Muntengwa of Njelele, Venda, South Africa is reported to be now 137 (26 September 1874)

Sweden

Swedish death registers contain detailed information on thousands of centenarians going back to 1749; the maximum age at death reported between 1751 and 1800 was 127.

• In 1689, Anna Persdotter in Leksand was said to have died at the age of 1024 years.

Switzerland Swiss anatomist Albrecht von Haller collected examples of 62 people ages 110–120, 29 ages 120–130, and 15 ages 130–140.

Turkey

• Halime Olcay (1 July 1874) Practices Diets The idea that certain diets can lead to extraordinary longevity (ages beyond 130) is not new.

In 1909, Elie Metchnikoff believed that drinking goat's milk could confer extraordinary longevity.

The Hunza diet, which has been claimed to give people the ability to live to 140 or more. There has been no proof that any diet has led humans to live longer than the genetically-recognized maximum (currently the oldest verified person, Jeanne Calment, died at age 122.45 years), however Caloric restriction diets have increased lifespans of rodents significantly.

Alchemy Traditions that have been believed to confer greater human longevity include alchemy. Nicolas Flamel (early 1330s – 1418?) was a 14th-century scrivener who developed a reputation as alchemist and creator of an "elixir of life" that conferred immortality upon himself and his wife Perenelle. His arcanely inscribed tombstone is preserved at the Musée de Cluny in Paris.

• Fridericus (Ludovicus) Gualdus, author of "Revelation of the True Chemical Wisdom", lived in Venice in the 1680s. His age was reported in a letter in a contemporary Dutch newspaper to be over 400. By some accounts, when asked about a portrait he carried, he said it was of himself, painted by Titian (who died in 1576), but gave no explanation and left Venice the following morning.

By another account, Gualdus left Venice due to religious accusations and died in 1724. The "Compass der Weisen" alludes to him as still alive in 1782 and nearly 600 years old.

Fountain of Youth Main article: Fountain of Youth. The Fountain of Youth reputedly restores the youth of anyone who drinks of its waters.

The New Testament, following older Jewish tradition, attributes healing to the Pool of Bethesda when the waters are "stirred" by an angel.

Herodotus attributes exceptional longevity to a fountain in the land of the Ethiopians.

The lore of the Alexander Romance and of Al-Khidr describes such a fountain, and stories about the philosopher's stone, universal panaceas, and the elixir of life are widespread.

After the death of Juan Ponce de León, Gonzalo Fernández de Oviedo wrote in Historia General y Natural de las Indias (1535) that Ponce de León was looking for the waters of Bimini to cure his aging.

Summary

In this book I've tried to provide all of the relevant materials from the course although not in the original video format. Many pictures are missing too.

Many of the records of long lived people are un-verified but I ask the question-how could you verify people well over one hundred years when birth certificates were not issued or not available?

I hope you got a lot out of this book towards a full understanding of the first principle of the 10 Principles of Personal Longevity and that the next training courses in this series will also be just as informative.

Marty Ettington

October 2018

www.ingramcontent.com/pod-product-compliance
Lightning Source LLC
Chambersburg PA
CBHW051217250726
48655CB00006B/2450